ORTHOPEDIC SURGERY RECOVERY COOKBOOK

A Comprehensive Guide To Optimal Surgery Recovery Nutrition, Featuring Healing Recipes, Meal Plans, And Expert Tips For Long-Term Wellness

DR. ALLAN FREDA

Contents

CHAPTER 1 10

NUTRITIONAL FOUNDATIONS FOR HEALING............12

Understanding the Role of Nutrition in Recovery 12

Essential Nutrients for Healing 13

Components of a Well-Balanced Diet........................14

Incorporating Superfoods for Optimal Healing 15

CHAPTER 2 17

PREPARING YOUR KITCHEN FOR RECOVERY.............17

Kitchen Tools and Gadgets to Make Cooking Easier:...18

Meal Planning Strategies for Success:..........................19

Simplifying Meal Prep for Busy Days: 20

CHAPTER 3 22

NOURISHING BREAKFASTS.....................................22

Nourishing Breakfasts:...23

3.3 Healing Porridges and Oatmeal Varieties: 25

CHAPTER 4 29

HEALING SOUPS AND SATISFYING SALADS.................29

Comforting Soups for Soothing Recovery.....................29

Wholesome Broths and Stocks 30

Filling Salads Packed with Nutrients and Flavor..........31

Dressings and Vinaigrettes to Enhance Your Salad
Experience..32

CHAPTER 5 34

EASY-TO-DIGEST MAIN COURSES 34

Tender Proteins for Gentle Chewing...........................34

Flavorful Vegetarian and Vegan Options 35

Simple One-Pot Meals for Minimal Cleanup 36

Incorporating Whole Grains for Sustained Energy 37

CHAPTER 6 38

NOURISHING SIDES AND SNACKS 38

Satisfying Vegetable Dishes 39

Crunchy and Creamy Snacks for Anytime Nibbles 40

Portable Snack Ideas for On-the-Go Healing 41

CHAPTER 7 44

DESSERTS AND TREATS FOR RECOVERY 44

Nutrient-Dense Treats for Occasional Indulgences 45

Creative Ways to Enjoy Fruits and Berries 46

DIY Energy Bars and Bites for Quick Energy Boosts 47

CHAPTER 8 49

HYDRATION AND HEALING BEVERAGES 49

Importance of Hydration During Recovery 49

Herbal Teas and Infusions for Relaxation and Healing
.... 50

Nutrient-Packed Smoothies for Easy Consumption 51

DIY Electrolyte Drinks for Replenishing Lost Nutrients
.... 52

CHAPTER 9 55

SPECIAL CONSIDERATIONS FOR ORTHOPEDIC
SURGERY RECOVERY 55

Managing Pain and Inflammation Through Diet 56

Dietary Tips for Bone Health and Strength 57

Supporting Healing Through Proper Nutrition 59

CHAPTER 10...65

BEYOND THE PLATE: HOLISTIC HEALING PRACTICES

....65

Mindful Eating for Enhanced Recovery: 66

Gentle Movement and Exercise During Rehabilitation:

....68

Stress Management Techniques for Overall Well-Being:

....70

CONCLUSION 75

Welcome to the comprehensive guide to optimal post-surgery diet for orthopedic surgery recovery. Following orthopedic surgery, proper nutrition plays a vital role in facilitating healing, reducing inflammation, and restoring strength and mobility. In this guide, we'll delve into the essential dietary considerations for individuals undergoing orthopedic surgery, providing healing recipes, meal plans, and expert tips for long-term wellness.

Understanding the Role of Nutrition in Orthopedic Surgery Recovery

Nutrition serves as a cornerstone in the recovery process following orthopedic surgery. Adequate nutrient intake is crucial for promoting tissue repair, supporting immune function, and preventing complications such as infections and delayed wound healing. Moreover, specific nutrients play key roles in bone health, muscle regeneration, and overall recovery.

Therefore, tailoring your diet to meet your body's increased nutritional needs during the recovery period is essential for optimizing outcomes and enhancing your overall well-being.

A Comprehensive Guide to Optimal Post-Surgery Diet

Nutritional Requirements for Orthopedic Surgery Recovery

Before delving into specific dietary recommendations, it's important to understand the nutritional requirements during orthopedic surgery recovery. Following surgery, the body's metabolic rate increases as it works to repair tissues and combat inflammation. This heightened metabolic demand necessitates adequate energy intake to fuel the healing process. Additionally, certain nutrients such as protein, vitamins, and minerals are particularly important for supporting tissue repair, reducing inflammation, and promoting bone health.

Therefore, a well-balanced diet rich in these essential nutrients is essential for optimal recovery.

Healing Recipes for Orthopedic Surgery Recovery

Incorporating healing recipes into your post-surgery diet can help provide the necessary nutrients to support recovery while satisfying your taste buds.

When preparing meals, focus on incorporating nutrient-dense foods such as lean proteins, whole grains, fruits, vegetables, and healthy fats. Additionally, consider incorporating ingredients known for their anti-inflammatory and healing properties, such as turmeric, ginger, garlic, and omega-3 fatty acids. Experimenting with different recipes and flavors can make the recovery process more enjoyable while ensuring you're meeting your nutritional needs.

Creating a structured meal plan can help ensure you're consistently meeting your nutritional requirements throughout the recovery period. When planning meals, aim for a balanced combination of macronutrients, including carbohydrates, proteins, and fats, to provide sustained energy and support tissue repair. Incorporate a variety of foods from each food group to ensure you're receiving a wide range of nutrients. Additionally, consider spacing out meals and snacks evenly throughout the day to maintain stable blood sugar levels and support optimal energy levels.

Expert Tips for Long-Term Wellness

In addition to focusing on immediate post-surgery recovery, it's important to adopt long-term dietary habits that support overall health and wellness. Incorporating a diverse range of nutrient-rich foods into your diet regularly can help promote optimal bone health, muscle strength, and joint function. Additionally, maintaining a healthy weight through balanced nutrition and regular physical activity can reduce the risk of orthopedic issues and support long-term joint health.

Consulting with a registered dietitian or nutritionist can provide personalized guidance and support in developing a sustainable dietary plan tailored to your specific needs and goals.

Optimizing nutrition plays a critical role in promoting recovery and enhancing overall well-being following orthopedic surgery. By focusing on nutrient-rich foods, incorporating healing recipes, following structured meal plans, and adopting long-term dietary habits, you can support your body's healing process and achieve optimal outcomes. Remember to consult with your healthcare provider or a registered dietitian for personalized guidance and support throughout your recovery journey. With dedication to proper nutrition and a focus on holistic wellness, you can navigate your orthopedic surgery recovery with confidence and resilience.

Disclaimer

The information in this book is for informational purposes only and should not replace professional medical advice, diagnosis, or treatment. Always consult your physician or a qualified health provider regarding any medical concerns. Do not disregard professional medical advice or delay seeking it based on information in this book.

The author does not endorse or have affiliations with any mentioned entities. References are for informational purposes only.

Consult your healthcare provider before making dietary or lifestyle changes, especially during recovery from surgery, as individual needs vary.

Results may vary, and the information provided is not guaranteed to produce specific outcomes.

By reading this book, you acknowledge and agree to consult your healthcare provider before implementing any information herein.

For further guidance, consult your healthcare provider or reputable medical websites for reliable information on surgery recovery diets.

CHAPTER 1
NUTRITIONAL FOUNDATIONS FOR HEALING

Nutrition plays a pivotal role in the recovery process after orthopedic surgery, serving as a cornerstone for optimal healing and rehabilitation. Understanding the intricate relationship between nutrition and recovery is essential for patients undergoing orthopedic procedures to achieve successful outcomes. This comprehensive guide aims to elucidate the fundamental concepts of nutrition in post-surgery recovery, emphasizing the importance of essential nutrients, balanced diet principles, and the integration of superfoods for expedited healing.

Understanding the Role of Nutrition in Recovery

In the realm of orthopedic surgery recovery, nutrition catalyzes the body's innate healing mechanisms.

Adequate nutrition not only fuels cellular repair and regeneration but also bolsters the immune system, mitigates inflammation, and supports overall physiological functions critical for recuperation. Following surgery, the body undergoes significant metabolic shifts and heightened nutrient demands to facilitate tissue repair and combat potential complications.

Thus, optimizing nutritional intake becomes paramount to enhance the efficacy of surgical interventions and promote optimal recovery outcomes.

Essential Nutrients for Healing

Several key nutrients play indispensable roles in the healing process following orthopedic surgery. Protein, often hailed as the building block of tissues, is particularly crucial for repairing damaged muscles, ligaments, and bones. Additionally, adequate intake of vitamins and minerals, such as vitamin C, vitamin D, calcium, and zinc, is essential for collagen synthesis, bone remineralization, and immune function, thereby accelerating the healing trajectory. Omega-3 fatty acids exhibit potent anti-inflammatory properties, which can alleviate postoperative inflammation and pain, facilitating rehabilitation. Furthermore, hydration remains paramount to maintain cellular function, support nutrient transport, and promote tissue hydration, all of which are critical for optimal recovery.

Crafting a well-rounded diet is imperative for supporting the intricate healing processes post-orthopedic surgery. A balanced diet encompasses a diverse array of nutrient-dense foods, including lean proteins, whole grains, fruits, vegetables, and healthy fats. Emphasizing lean protein sources, such as poultry, fish, tofu, and legumes, ensures an ample supply of amino acids necessary for tissue repair and muscle regeneration. Whole grains provide sustained energy release and essential micronutrients, while fruits and vegetables offer an abundance of vitamins, minerals, and antioxidants crucial for immune support and tissue healing. Incorporating healthy fats from sources like avocados, nuts, seeds, and olive oil aids in inflammation modulation and cellular membrane integrity, fostering an optimal environment for recovery.

Superfoods, revered for their exceptional nutrient density and health-promoting properties, can serve as valuable allies in the orthopedic surgery recovery journey. Berries, such as blueberries, strawberries, and raspberries, boast potent antioxidant compounds that combat oxidative stress and inflammation, bolstering tissue repair mechanisms. Dark leafy greens like spinach, kale, and Swiss chard are rich in vitamins K and C, calcium, and magnesium, all of which are pivotal for bone health and fracture healing. Turmeric, renowned for its anti-inflammatory curcumin compound, can help alleviate postoperative pain and swelling, expediting the rehabilitation process.

Additionally, incorporating omega-3-rich foods like salmon, chia seeds, and walnuts can further enhance the anti-inflammatory milieu, facilitating a smoother recovery trajectory.

nutrition serves as a cornerstone for optimal healing and recovery following orthopedic surgery. By understanding the critical role of essential nutrients, adhering to the principles of a balanced diet, and integrating superfoods into one's meal plan, patients can expedite the healing process, minimize complications, and promote long-term wellness. As such, personalized nutritional strategies tailored to individual needs and surgical requirements are integral components of comprehensive orthopedic care, ensuring successful outcomes and improved quality of life for patients undergoing surgical interventions.

CHAPTER 2
PREPARING YOUR KITCHEN FOR RECOVERY

Ensuring your kitchen is adequately stocked and equipped is essential for a smooth and successful recovery from orthopedic surgery. A well-prepared kitchen not only facilitates the healing process but also makes meal preparation more manageable, especially during times when mobility may be limited. Here's a comprehensive guide to help you prepare your kitchen for optimal post-surgery recovery.

Stocking Your Pantry with Recovery-Friendly Ingredients:

Stocking your pantry with recovery-friendly ingredients is fundamental to supporting your healing journey.

Opt for nutrient-dense foods that promote tissue repair, reduce inflammation, and boost overall health.

Include plenty of lean proteins such as chicken, fish, tofu, and legumes to support muscle recovery and strength. Incorporate whole grains like quinoa, brown rice, and oats for sustained energy levels and fiber to aid digestion. Additionally, ensure your pantry is filled with a variety of fruits and vegetables rich in vitamins, minerals, and antioxidants to support immune function and tissue healing. Consider incorporating healthy fats such as olive oil, nuts, and seeds to reduce inflammation and support heart health. Lastly, stock up on herbs, spices, and condiments to add flavor to your meals without compromising on nutrition.

Kitchen Tools and Gadgets to Make Cooking Easier:
Investing in kitchen tools and gadgets can significantly simplify the cooking process, especially when mobility is limited post-surgery.

Consider purchasing ergonomic utensils and gadgets designed to reduce strain on your joints and muscles, such as lightweight knives with easy-grip handles and ergonomic vegetable peelers.

A food processor or blender can be invaluable for chopping, pureeing, and blending ingredients, making it easier to prepare nutritious meals with minimal effort. Additionally, consider using kitchen appliances like slow cookers, Instant Pots, or air fryers that require minimal supervision and effort to prepare delicious and healthy meals.

Stock your kitchen with non-stick cookware and baking sheets to minimize the need for excessive oil and make cleaning up a breeze. Having these tools readily available can make cooking more accessible and enjoyable during your recovery period.

Meal Planning Strategies for Success:
Effective meal planning is key to ensuring you have nutritious and balanced meals readily

available throughout your recovery period. Start by creating a weekly meal plan that includes a variety of protein sources, whole grains, fruits, vegetables, and healthy fats to meet your nutritional needs. Consider preparing large batches of meals in advance and freezing them in individual portions for easy reheating when needed. Utilize leftovers creatively by incorporating them into salads, sandwiches, or stir-fries to minimize food waste and save time in the kitchen. Experiment with different cuisines and recipes to keep meals interesting and flavorful, but make sure they align with your dietary restrictions and nutritional goals. Additionally, involve family members or friends in meal planning and preparation to lighten the load and foster a sense of community support during your recovery journey.

Simplifying Meal Prep for Busy Days:
On busy days when time and energy are limited, simplifying meal prep can help ensure you still have access to nutritious meals without added

stress. Consider utilizing convenience foods like pre-cut vegetables, pre-cooked grains, and canned beans to streamline meal preparation and minimize cooking time. Batch cooking on days when you have more energy can also be beneficial – prepare large quantities of staple ingredients like grains, proteins, and roasted vegetables that can be easily assembled into different meals throughout the week.

Make use of meal delivery services or grocery delivery apps to have fresh ingredients and prepared meals delivered to your doorstep, saving you time and energy on grocery shopping and meal preparation. Additionally, don't hesitate to enlist the help of family members, friends, or caregivers to assist with meal prep or household chores during times when you're feeling overwhelmed or fatigued.

By simplifying meal prep and enlisting support when needed, you can ensure that your nutritional needs are met even on the busiest of days during your recovery period.

CHAPTER 3
NOURISHING BREAKFASTS

Orthopedic surgery is a critical medical intervention aimed at correcting musculoskeletal issues, such as fractures, joint injuries, and degenerative conditions. Recovery from orthopedic surgery is a multifaceted process that involves not only physical rehabilitation but also comprehensive nutritional support. Proper nutrition plays a crucial role in promoting healing, reducing inflammation, and supporting overall health during the recovery period. In this guide, we will delve into the importance of nourishing breakfasts in orthopedic surgery recovery, exploring energizing smoothies and shakes, protein-packed breakfast bowls, healing porridges, and creative egg dishes as essential components of a post-surgery diet.

Breakfast is often hailed as the most important meal of the day, and this holds especially true for individuals recovering from orthopedic surgery.

A nourishing breakfast sets the tone for the rest of the day, providing essential nutrients and energy to support healing and recovery. Incorporating a variety of nutrient-dense foods into breakfast can help optimize healing, promote muscle repair, and enhance overall well-being. In the following sections, we will explore different breakfast options specifically tailored to support orthopedic surgery recovery.

3.1 Energizing Smoothies and Shakes:

Energizing smoothies and shakes are excellent breakfast options for individuals recovering from orthopedic surgery. These beverages are not only convenient and easy to digest but also packed with essential nutrients that support healing and recovery.

A well-balanced smoothie or shake typically includes a combination of fruits, vegetables, protein sources, healthy fats, and additional supplements as needed. Ingredients such as leafy greens, berries, bananas, Greek yogurt, nut butter, and protein powder can be blended to create delicious and nutritious breakfast options. Incorporating ingredients rich in antioxidants, vitamins, and minerals can help reduce inflammation, boost immune function, and promote tissue repair, making smoothies and shakes an ideal choice for orthopedic surgery recovery.

3.2 Protein-Packed Breakfast Bowls:

Protein is an essential nutrient for individuals recovering from orthopedic surgery as it plays a crucial role in tissue repair and muscle regeneration. Protein-packed breakfast bowls offer a convenient and versatile way to incorporate high-quality protein sources into the morning meal. Ingredients such as eggs, lean meats, fish, tofu, beans, and quinoa can be combined with vegetables, grains, and healthy fats to create delicious and satisfying breakfast bowls.

Adding toppings such as avocado, nuts, seeds, and Greek yogurt can further enhance the protein content and nutritional value of the meal. Consuming a protein-rich breakfast can help promote muscle recovery, prevent muscle loss, and support overall strength and mobility during the recovery process.

3.3 Healing Porridges and Oatmeal Varieties:
Porridges and oatmeal varieties are classic breakfast options that provide comfort, warmth, and nourishment, making them particularly suitable for individuals recovering from orthopedic surgery. These hearty breakfast dishes are rich in complex carbohydrates, fiber, and essential

nutrients that help sustain energy levels and promote satiety throughout the morning.

Additionally, oatmeal is known for its anti-inflammatory properties, which can help reduce swelling and discomfort associated with surgery.

By incorporating ingredients such as rolled oats, almond milk, fruits, nuts, and spices, individuals can create flavorful and nutritious porridges and oatmeal varieties that support healing and recovery. Adding ingredients like cinnamon, turmeric, and ginger can further enhance the anti-inflammatory properties of these breakfast dishes, making them an excellent choice for orthopedic surgery recovery.

3.4 Creative Egg Dishes for Morning Fuel:

Eggs are a versatile and nutrient-dense food that can be incorporated into a variety of creative breakfast dishes to support orthopedic surgery recovery. Eggs are an excellent source of high-quality protein, vitamins, minerals, and antioxidants, making them an ideal choice for promoting healing and recovery. Creative egg dishes such as omelettes, frittatas, and egg muffins offer a delicious and convenient way to enjoy the nutritional benefits of eggs while incorporating additional ingredients for flavor and variety. Ingredients such as vegetables, cheese, herbs, and lean meats can be added to egg dishes to enhance their nutrient content and provide essential nutrients that support healing.

Consuming egg-based breakfast dishes can help increase protein intake, support muscle repair, and enhance overall nutritional status during the recovery period.

nourishing breakfasts play a crucial role in supporting orthopedic surgery recovery by providing essential nutrients, promoting healing, and enhancing overall well-being. Incorporating energizing smoothies and shakes, protein-packed breakfast bowls, healing porridges, and creative egg dishes into the morning meal can help optimize nutritional intake and support the recovery process. By choosing nutrient-dense foods and incorporating a variety of flavors and textures, individuals can create delicious and satisfying breakfast options that contribute to long-term wellness and vitality during the rehabilitation journey.

CHAPTER 4
HEALING SOUPS AND SATISFYING SALADS

After undergoing orthopedic surgery, a crucial aspect of the recovery process involves dietary choices that promote healing, boost immunity, and provide essential nutrients for tissue repair. In this section, we delve into the significance of incorporating healing soups and satisfying salads into your post-surgery diet regimen.

From comforting soups for soothing recovery to wholesome broths and stocks, along with filling salads packed with nutrients and flavor, we explore how these culinary choices can optimize your healing journey.

Comforting Soups for Soothing Recovery

During the post-surgery period, when the body is in a state of recovery, comforting soups serve as an excellent option for providing nourishment without taxing the digestive system.

These soups are often rich in vitamins, minerals, and antioxidants, which are essential for supporting the body's immune function and promoting tissue repair. Ingredients such as root vegetables, leafy greens, lean proteins, and whole grains can be incorporated into soups to enhance their nutritional value. Additionally, the warmth of soups can have a soothing effect on the throat and digestive tract, making them particularly beneficial for individuals experiencing discomfort or difficulty swallowing post-surgery. Incorporating a variety of herbs and spices not only enhances the flavor profile but also provides anti-inflammatory and antimicrobial properties, further supporting the healing process.

Wholesome Broths and Stocks

Broths and stocks form the foundation of many healing soups and are renowned for their nutritional benefits.

Rich in collagen, amino acids, and minerals such as calcium, magnesium, and phosphorus, these liquid bases provide essential nutrients that promote bone health and tissue regeneration.

Whether homemade or store-bought, opting for low-sodium varieties ensures that you receive the maximum nutritional value without excessive salt intake, which can potentially interfere with the healing process. Additionally, the versatility of broths and stocks allows for customization according to individual preferences and dietary restrictions. Vegetarian alternatives, such as mushroom or vegetable broth, offer a flavorful option for those adhering to plant-based diets while still providing ample nutrients to support recovery.

Filling Salads Packed with Nutrients and Flavor

While soups are often favored for their comforting nature, salads offer a refreshing and nutrient-dense alternative that can complement your post-surgery diet. Filling salads packed with a variety of colorful vegetables, lean proteins, healthy fats, and whole grains provide a diverse array of nutrients essential for healing and overall well-being. Incorporating ingredients such as leafy greens, cruciferous vegetables, avocado, nuts, seeds, and lean proteins like grilled chicken or tofu not only adds texture and flavor but also ensures a balanced and satisfying meal. Moreover, salads are an excellent way to increase your intake of fiber, antioxidants, and phytonutrients, which play a crucial role in reducing inflammation, supporting immune function, and promoting tissue repair. Experimenting with different combinations of ingredients and dressings allows for endless possibilities, catering to individual taste preferences and dietary needs.

Dressings and Vinaigrettes to Enhance Your Salad Experience

The key to elevating the flavor profile of salads lies in the dressings and vinaigrettes used to enhance their taste and texture. Opting for homemade dressings allows for greater control over the ingredients, ensuring that they align with your dietary goals and preferences. Incorporating heart-healthy oils such as olive oil, avocado oil, or flaxseed oil as the base provides essential fatty acids that support inflammation regulation and promote cardiovascular health.

Adding acidic components such as lemon juice, balsamic vinegar, or apple cider vinegar not only enhances the flavor but also aids in digestion and nutrient absorption. Herbs, spices, and aromatics such as garlic, ginger, fresh herbs, and citrus zest can be used to add depth and complexity to the dressing while providing additional health benefits. Experimenting with different flavor combinations allows for versatility and creativity, ensuring that your salads remain enjoyable and satisfying throughout your recovery journey.

CHAPTER 5
EASY-TO-DIGEST MAIN COURSES

After orthopedic surgery, a crucial aspect of the recovery process is maintaining a balanced and nutritious diet. This is essential not only for the body to heal efficiently but also to support overall health and well-being. The main courses consumed during recovery should be easy to digest, providing the necessary nutrients without putting unnecessary strain on the digestive system. In this section, we will delve into various options for main courses that are gentle on the stomach and promote healing post-surgery.

Tender Proteins for Gentle Chewing

Proteins are vital for tissue repair and muscle rebuilding, making them indispensable during the recovery phase after orthopedic surgery. However, for individuals with limited jaw mobility or discomfort while chewing, opting for tender proteins is paramount. These include options such as poached or baked fish, shredded chicken or turkey, tofu, and eggs. These protein sources are soft and easy to chew, minimizing discomfort while still providing the necessary amino acids for healing. Incorporating these tender proteins into main courses ensures that patients receive adequate nutrition without exacerbating post-operative challenges.

For individuals following a vegetarian or vegan diet, there is a plethora of flavorful options available to meet their nutritional needs during orthopedic surgery recovery. Plant-based proteins such as lentils, beans, chickpeas, and quinoa are excellent sources of protein and other essential nutrients. Main courses featuring these ingredients can include hearty salads, vegetable stir-fries, bean-based stews, and quinoa bowls. Additionally, incorporating a variety of herbs, spices, and flavorful sauces enhances the taste and enjoyment of these dishes without compromising on nutritional value. By embracing vegetarian and vegan options, patients can optimize their recovery while adhering to their dietary preferences.

During the recovery period, it's essential to minimize stress and fatigue, including when it comes to meal preparation and cleanup. One-pot meals offer a convenient solution, requiring minimal effort and cleanup while still delivering nourishing and satisfying main courses.

These meals typically involve combining protein, carbohydrates, and vegetables in a single pot or pan, resulting in a wholesome and balanced dish. Examples of one-pot meals suitable for orthopedic surgery recovery include vegetable and chicken soup, quinoa and vegetable skillet, and lentil stew. Not only are these meals easy to prepare, but they also provide a diverse array of nutrients necessary for healing and overall well-being.

Whole grains are an essential component of a post-surgery diet, providing sustained energy and essential nutrients such as fiber, vitamins, and minerals. Incorporating whole grains into main courses ensures that patients receive the necessary nutrients for recovery while promoting digestive health and satiety. Options such as brown rice, quinoa, barley, and whole wheat pasta can serve as the foundation for nutritious and satisfying main dishes. Pairing these grains with lean proteins, vegetables, and healthy fats creates well-rounded meals that support healing and long-term wellness. By prioritizing whole grains in main courses, patients can optimize their recovery and maintain energy levels throughout the rehabilitation process.

CHAPTER 6
NOURISHING SIDES AND SNACKS

Orthopedic surgery recovery is a critical phase in the journey toward restoring musculoskeletal health and functionality.

It involves a multifaceted approach encompassing medical care, physical therapy, and lifestyle adjustments. Central to successful recovery is the implementation of an optimal post-surgery diet, which plays a pivotal role in promoting healing, combating inflammation, and supporting overall well-being.

This comprehensive guide delves into the nuances of crafting a nourishing diet tailored to individuals navigating orthopedic surgery recovery. From featuring healing recipes to offering meal plans and expert tips, this guide aims to empower patients with the knowledge and resources necessary for long-term wellness.

In the realm of orthopedic surgery recovery, integrating a plethora of nutrient-rich vegetables into one's diet is paramount. Vegetables serve as powerhouse sources of vitamins, minerals, and antioxidants essential for tissue repair and immune function. Crafting satisfying vegetable dishes not only ensures adequate nutrient intake but also adds variety and flavor to meals, enhancing overall enjoyment. Incorporating a diverse array of colorful vegetables such as leafy greens, bell peppers, carrots, and broccoli can provide a spectrum of nutrients crucial for healing and recovery.

From roasted root vegetables to vibrant salads, the possibilities for vegetable-based dishes are endless. Additionally, cooking methods such as steaming, roasting, or stir-frying can help preserve the nutritional integrity of vegetables while enhancing their taste and texture.

During orthopedic surgery recovery, having convenient and nutritious snack options readily available is essential for maintaining energy levels and supporting healing processes. Crunchy and creamy snacks offer a satisfying combination of textures while providing a dose of essential nutrients. Nuts and seeds, such as almonds, walnuts, and pumpkin seeds, are excellent sources of healthy fats, protein, and micronutrients, making them ideal for snacking. Pairing nuts with sliced fruits or vegetables adds freshness and variety to snacks while increasing their nutrient density. Similarly, creamy snacks like Greek yogurt or hummus provide protein, probiotics, and satiating fats, promoting muscle repair and gut health. Incorporating whole grain crackers, rice cakes, or vegetable sticks for dipping adds crunch and fiber, enhancing the nutritional profile of snacks.

Maintaining nourishment and hydration while on the go is crucial for individuals undergoing orthopedic surgery recovery, especially during appointments, physical therapy sessions, or daily activities. Portable snack ideas offer convenience without compromising nutritional quality, ensuring continuous support for the healing process.

Preparing a homemade trail mix with a combination of nuts, dried fruits, and whole-grain cereals provides a balanced blend of carbohydrates, protein, and healthy fats for sustained energy. Additionally, pre-portioned snacks such as energy bars, fruit slices, or cheese sticks are easy to pack and consume on the move.

For a refreshing option, preparing fruit and vegetable smoothies or protein shakes in advance allows for quick and nourishing on-the-go snacks. Investing in reusable containers or insulated lunch bags can help keep snacks fresh and accessible throughout the day.

Dips, Spreads, and Sauces to Elevate Your Sides and Snacks

Enhancing the flavor and nutritional value of sides and snacks can be achieved through the incorporation of wholesome dips, spreads, and sauces. These culinary additions not only add depth and complexity to meals but also provide additional nutrients and hydration.

Hummus, guacamole, and tzatziki are versatile dips rich in healthy fats, protein, and fiber, perfect for pairing with vegetable sticks or whole-grain crackers.

Nut butter spreads, such as almond or cashew butter, offer a creamy texture and a boost of protein and essential fats, ideal for spreading on toast or fruit slices. Additionally, incorporating homemade sauces like pesto, salsa, or tahini dressing can elevate the taste of salads, wraps, or grain bowls while providing a burst of flavor and nutrients. Experimenting with herbs, spices, and citrus juices can further enhance the aroma and nutritional profile of dips, spreads, and sauces, making them indispensable components of a well-rounded post-surgery diet.

CHAPTER 7

DESSERTS AND TREATS FOR RECOVERY

When focusing on orthopedic surgery recovery, a crucial yet often overlooked aspect is nutrition.

A comprehensive post-surgery diet can significantly impact the healing process, ensuring optimal recovery and long-term wellness. Desserts and treats play a role in this diet, providing not only enjoyment but also essential nutrients to aid in the healing process. In this section, we'll explore various options for guilt-free desserts, nutrient-dense treats, creative fruit-based options, and homemade energy bars and bites designed to support recovery and overall well-being.

Guilt-Free Desserts to Satisfy Your Sweet Tooth

Guilt-free desserts offer a delightful way to indulge without compromising on nutritional quality.

These treats are typically low in added sugars, unhealthy fats, and processed ingredients, making them suitable for individuals recovering from orthopedic surgery. Options such as fruit sorbets, yogurt parfaits with fresh berries, and homemade fruit popsicles provide sweetness without excessive calories or artificial additives. Incorporating whole grains, nuts, and seeds into dessert recipes can also boost fiber and protein content, aiding in satiety and promoting healing.

Nutrient-Dense Treats for Occasional Indulgences

While indulging in desserts is permissible, it's essential to prioritize nutrient density, especially during the recovery phase. Nutrient-dense treats offer a balance between satisfaction and health benefits, supplying essential vitamins, minerals, and antioxidants. Dark chocolate-covered almonds or strawberries provide a satisfying crunch along with heart-healthy fats and antioxidants. Greek yogurt topped with honey and sliced almonds offers a protein-rich option that supports muscle repair and recovery.

Incorporating superfoods like chia seeds or flaxseeds into dessert recipes adds omega-3 fatty acids and fiber, promoting inflammation reduction and gastrointestinal health.

Creative Ways to Enjoy Fruits and Berries

Fruits and berries are natural sources of vitamins, minerals, and phytonutrients, making them ideal for enhancing post-surgery recovery. Creative preparations can elevate their appeal while maximizing nutritional benefits. Grilled peaches drizzled with a touch of honey and sprinkled with cinnamon offer a warm and comforting dessert option packed with vitamin C and fiber.

Berry smoothie bowls topped with granola and shredded coconut provide a refreshing treat loaded with antioxidants and essential nutrients. Incorporating fruits into baked goods, such as banana oat cookies or mixed berry muffins made with whole grain flour, offers a healthier alternative to traditional desserts while still satisfying cravings.

DIY Energy Bars and Bites for Quick Energy Boosts

Energy bars and bites are convenient snacks that can provide quick energy boosts during the recovery period. Crafting homemade versions allows for customization and ensures the use of wholesome ingredients. A base of oats, nuts, and dates blended forms the foundation for various flavor combinations. Adding ingredients like dried fruits, coconut flakes, and cocoa powder enhances taste while providing essential nutrients.

Protein-rich options, such as peanut butter or hemp seeds, contribute to muscle repair and satiety.

These homemade energy bars and bites can be portioned and stored for easy access, making them perfect for busy days or as pre- or post-workout snacks to support recovery and sustained energy levels.

Incorporating a variety of guilt-free desserts, nutrient-dense treats, fruit-based options, and homemade energy bars and bites into the post-surgery diet can enhance recovery outcomes and promote long-term wellness. By focusing on quality ingredients and balanced nutrition, individuals undergoing orthopedic surgery can enjoy satisfying treats while supporting their bodies' healing processes. Consulting with a healthcare professional or registered dietitian can help tailor dietary recommendations to individual needs and ensure optimal recovery and overall health.

CHAPTER 8
<u>HYDRATION AND HEALING</u>
<u>BEVERAGES</u>

Ensuring adequate hydration is paramount during the recovery phase following orthopedic surgery. Proper hydration supports cellular function, facilitates nutrient transport, aids in the elimination of toxins, and maintains overall bodily functions. In the context of orthopedic surgery recovery, where the body undergoes significant stress and repair, maintaining optimal hydration levels becomes even more crucial. Let's delve into the importance of hydration during recovery and explore various healing beverages that can aid in the process.

Importance of Hydration During Recovery

Hydration plays a pivotal role in the body's ability to heal after orthopedic surgery. Surgery induces physiological stress, triggering inflammation and increasing metabolic demands.

Adequate hydration supports these processes by ensuring efficient delivery of nutrients to cells, facilitating tissue repair and regeneration. Furthermore, proper hydration promotes optimal blood circulation, reducing the risk of complications such as blood clots, which are particularly concerning during periods of limited mobility post-surgery. Dehydration, on the other hand, can impede healing, prolong recovery times, and increase susceptibility to infections. Therefore, maintaining adequate hydration levels through the consumption of water and other hydrating beverages is essential for supporting the body's recovery journey.

Herbal Teas and Infusions for Relaxation and Healing

Herbal teas and infusions offer a soothing and therapeutic way to hydrate during the recovery process. Certain herbs possess anti-inflammatory, analgesic, and calming properties that can aid in alleviating post-operative discomfort and promoting relaxation, which is crucial for facilitating healing. Chamomile tea, for example, contains compounds that have been shown to reduce inflammation and promote sleep quality, supporting the body's healing mechanisms.

Ginger tea is another beneficial option, known for its anti-nausea and anti-inflammatory effects, which can be particularly helpful in managing post-surgical nausea and discomfort. Additionally, herbal infusions such as peppermint or lavender can provide relief from muscle tension and promote relaxation, contributing to an overall sense of well-being during the recovery period.

Nutrient-Packed Smoothies for Easy Consumption

Nutrient-packed smoothies offer a convenient and easily digestible way to replenish vital nutrients during orthopedic surgery recovery.

Following surgery, appetite may be diminished, and consuming solid foods may be challenging initially. Smoothies provide a practical solution by combining nutrient-rich ingredients into a palatable and easy-to-consume form. Incorporating ingredients such as leafy greens, fruits, nuts, seeds, and protein sources like Greek yogurt or plant-based protein powder can ensure a diverse array of essential vitamins, minerals, antioxidants, and proteins necessary for tissue repair and immune function. Moreover, adding ingredients like avocado or coconut milk can provide healthy fats, which are crucial for cellular integrity and hormone production. Customizing smoothie recipes to include ingredients that target specific nutritional needs or symptoms, such as inflammation or fatigue, can further enhance their therapeutic value during the recovery process.

Electrolyte imbalance is a common concern during orthopedic surgery recovery, especially if there has been significant fluid loss through sweating, vomiting, or other factors.

Electrolytes such as sodium, potassium, calcium, and magnesium play essential roles in muscle function, nerve transmission, and fluid balance, all of which are critical for optimal recovery. DIY electrolyte drinks offer a practical and cost-effective way to replenish these lost nutrients and maintain electrolyte balance.

A basic recipe may include ingredients such as water, citrus juice for vitamin C and flavor, a pinch of sea salt for sodium and other minerals, and a natural sweetener like honey or maple syrup. Adding coconut water provides additional potassium and magnesium, while a splash of fruit juice can enhance taste and provide additional vitamins and antioxidants. Customizing electrolyte drinks to individual preferences and needs ensures optimal hydration and nutrient replenishment, supporting the body's recovery process effectively.

hydration and healing beverages play a vital role in supporting optimal recovery following orthopedic surgery. Adequate hydration facilitates cellular repair, nutrient delivery, and overall physiological function, while specific healing beverages such as herbal teas, nutrient-packed smoothies, and DIY electrolyte drinks offer additional therapeutic benefits. By incorporating these beverages into a comprehensive post-surgery diet plan, individuals can enhance their recovery experience, promote healing, and optimize long-term wellness.

CHAPTER 9
SPECIAL CONSIDERATIONS FOR ORTHOPEDIC SURGERY RECOVERY

Orthopedic surgery recovery is a multifaceted process that requires careful attention to various aspects of health and well-being. Beyond the surgical procedure itself, recovery involves managing pain, promoting healing, and optimizing overall nutrition to support the body's repair processes. In this comprehensive guide, we will delve into key considerations for orthopedic surgery recovery, including managing pain and inflammation through diet, tips for maintaining bone health and strength, the importance of proper nutrition in supporting healing, and addressing common digestive issues and concerns that may arise during the recovery period.

One of the primary challenges during orthopedic surgery recovery is managing pain and inflammation, which are natural responses to tissue trauma caused by the surgical procedure. While pain medications prescribed by healthcare professionals play a crucial role in alleviating discomfort, dietary interventions can also complement these efforts and contribute to overall pain management.

Certain foods have been found to possess anti-inflammatory properties, which can help reduce swelling and discomfort post-surgery.

Incorporating foods rich in omega-3 fatty acids, such as salmon, walnuts, and flaxseeds, into the diet can help mitigate inflammation and promote healing. These healthy fats are known for their anti-inflammatory effects and can aid in reducing postoperative pain. Additionally, consuming plenty of fruits and vegetables, particularly those high in antioxidants, such as berries, leafy greens, and citrus fruits, can further support the body's natural inflammatory response and enhance recovery.

Furthermore, it's essential to maintain proper hydration levels during recovery, as dehydration can exacerbate inflammation and prolong healing time. Opting for hydrating foods like watermelon, cucumber, and broth-based soups can help replenish fluids lost during surgery and promote tissue repair. Avoiding processed foods high in refined sugars and unhealthy fats is also advisable, as these can contribute to inflammation and hinder the recovery process.

Dietary Tips for Bone Health and Strength

Orthopedic surgery often involves procedures related to the musculoskeletal system, including bones, joints, and connective tissues. Therefore, maintaining optimal bone health and strength is paramount for successful recovery and long-term well-being. A diet rich in essential nutrients, such as calcium, vitamin D, and protein, plays a crucial role in supporting bone health and promoting healing after orthopedic surgery.

Calcium is a fundamental mineral required for bone formation and strength. Dairy products like milk, yogurt, and cheese are excellent sources of calcium, along with fortified plant-based alternatives like soy milk and tofu. Leafy greens such as kale, broccoli, and collard greens also contain calcium and can be incorporated into meals to boost bone health.

Vitamin D is essential for calcium absorption and bone mineralization, making it a vital nutrient for orthopedic surgery recovery. Exposure to sunlight is the primary source of vitamin D production in the body, but dietary sources such as fatty fish (e.g., salmon, mackerel), egg yolks, and fortified foods like orange juice and cereal can also contribute to vitamin D intake.

Additionally, protein plays a critical role in tissue repair and muscle maintenance, both of which are essential components of orthopedic surgery recovery.

Lean sources of protein such as poultry, fish, beans, lentils, and tofu should be included in post-surgery meals to support healing and optimize recovery outcomes.

Ensuring an adequate intake of these key nutrients through a well-balanced diet can help promote bone health, enhance strength, and facilitate the healing process following orthopedic surgery.

Proper nutrition is a cornerstone of orthopedic surgery recovery, as it provides the essential nutrients needed for tissue repair, immune function, and overall healing. In addition to specific dietary recommendations for managing pain, inflammation, and bone health, there are general principles of nutrition that can support the body's recovery efforts post-surgery.

First and foremost, it's essential to consume a well-rounded diet that includes a variety of nutrient-dense foods from all food groups. This ensures that the body receives the necessary vitamins, minerals, antioxidants, and macronutrients to support healing and optimize recovery outcomes.

Aim to include a rainbow of fruits and vegetables in your meals to maximize your intake of vitamins, minerals, and phytonutrients that promote healing and reduce inflammation. Incorporating whole grains such as brown rice, quinoa, and oats provides fiber, which aids in digestion and helps maintain stable blood sugar levels, crucial for energy production and overall well-being during recovery.

Healthy fats from sources like avocados, nuts, seeds, and olive oil are important for reducing inflammation and supporting cellular function. Including these fats in moderation can help optimize nutrient absorption and promote healing post-surgery.

Moreover, staying hydrated is essential for flushing out toxins, transporting nutrients, and maintaining overall health and vitality. Drink as much water as possible throughout the day, and include foods high in water content, such as fruits,

vegetables, and soups into your meals to support hydration and aid in the recovery process.

Lastly, listening to your body's hunger and fullness cues and eating mindfully can help ensure that you're nourishing yourself adequately during the recovery period. Pay attention to how different foods make you feel and adjust your diet accordingly to support your body's healing needs.

By focusing on proper nutrition and adopting healthy eating habits, you can support the healing process, optimize recovery outcomes, and promote long-term wellness following orthopedic surgery.

Addressing Digestive Issues and Common Concerns

Orthopedic surgery recovery can sometimes be accompanied by digestive issues and common concerns related to dietary changes, medication side effects, and decreased physical activity. Addressing these issues proactively through dietary modifications and lifestyle adjustments can help alleviate discomfort and support overall well-being during the recovery period.

One common concern during orthopedic surgery recovery is constipation, which can be exacerbated by pain medications, reduced mobility, and changes in diet. To promote regularity and prevent constipation, it's important to consume an adequate amount of fiber-rich foods such as fruits, vegetables, whole grains, and legumes. Additionally, staying hydrated by drinking plenty of water and herbal teas can help soften stools and facilitate bowel movements.

Another digestive issue that may arise post-surgery is nausea and vomiting, often as a side effect of anesthesia or pain medications.

Eating smaller, more frequent meals and avoiding heavy or greasy foods can help minimize these symptoms. Opting for bland, easily digestible foods like crackers, toast, bananas, and rice can also provide relief from nausea and support digestion.

Some individuals may experience changes in appetite or taste preferences during orthopedic surgery recovery, which can affect their dietary intake and nutritional status. Experimenting with different flavors, textures, and meal formats can help stimulate appetite and make eating more enjoyable. Including nutrient-dense foods that are easy to digest, such as smoothies, soups, and nutrient-rich snacks, can ensure that nutritional needs are met even when appetite is diminished.

Additionally, it's important to be mindful of potential food-drug interactions, particularly with pain medications and other medications prescribed during the recovery period. Certain foods and beverages may interact with medications, affecting their absorption, metabolism, or effectiveness. Consulting with healthcare professionals or pharmacists about potential food-drug interactions and adjusting your diet accordingly can help minimize adverse effects and support optimal recovery.

Overall, addressing digestive issues and common concerns related to diet and nutrition is an essential aspect of orthopedic surgery recovery. By making appropriate dietary modifications, staying hydrated, and being mindful of potential food-drug interactions, you can support digestive health and enhance overall well-being during the recovery process.

CHAPTER 10
BEYOND THE PLATE: HOLISTIC HEALING PRACTICES

Orthopedic surgery recovery is a critical period that requires comprehensive care to optimize healing and restore functionality. While medical interventions play a significant role in this process, holistic approaches that encompass mindful eating, gentle movement, stress management, and self-care can significantly enhance recovery outcomes. In this guide, we delve into these holistic healing practices to provide a comprehensive understanding of their importance and how they can be integrated into the post-surgery recovery journey.

Eating and drinking mindfully entails giving your entire attention to the process, both inside and outwardly.

It encompasses being present in the moment, acknowledging sensations such as hunger and satiety, and recognizing the flavors, textures, and smells of food. In the context of orthopedic surgery recovery, mindful eating can play a crucial role in facilitating optimal healing and overall well-being.

When recovering from orthopedic surgery, proper nutrition is essential for tissue repair, immune function, and energy production.

 Mindful eating can help individuals make healthier food choices by fostering awareness of their body's nutritional needs and preferences. By paying attention to hunger cues and satiety signals, individuals can avoid overeating or undereating, thus promoting a balanced diet that supports recovery.

Furthermore, mindful eating can enhance the enjoyment of food, even when dietary restrictions are present. By Savoring each bite and appreciating the flavors and textures of meals, individuals can derive greater satisfaction from their food choices, which can positively impact their overall mood and well-being during the recovery process.

Incorporating mindfulness practices such as deep breathing or meditation before meals can also help individuals cultivate a sense of calm and relaxation, reducing stress levels and promoting digestion. Additionally, being mindful of portion sizes and meal composition can support weight management goals, which may be particularly relevant for individuals with mobility limitations during recovery.

Overall, mindful eating is a powerful tool for promoting optimal nutrition, reducing stress, and enhancing the overall experience of food consumption during orthopedic surgery recovery. By integrating mindful eating practices into their daily routine, individuals can support their body's healing process and improve their overall quality of life.

Gentle movement and exercise are integral components of the rehabilitation process following orthopedic surgery. While it's essential to allow adequate time for tissues to heal, incorporating controlled movements and exercises under the guidance of a healthcare professional can promote flexibility, strength, and overall functionality.

During the initial stages of recovery, gentle movement exercises may focus on restoring range of motion and preventing stiffness in the affected joints or muscles. These exercises typically involve controlled movements within a pain-free range and may include activities such as gentle stretching, passive range-of-motion exercises, and low-impact activities like walking or swimming.

As the recovery progresses and tissues continue to heal, the focus of rehabilitation exercises may shift towards building strength and stability in the surrounding muscles and tissues. This may involve targeted exercises to improve muscle tone, balance, and coordination, as well as functional activities that mimic daily tasks and movements.

Individuals need to work closely with their healthcare team or a qualified physical therapist to develop a personalized exercise program tailored to their specific needs and recovery goals. A gradual progression of exercises, with careful monitoring of symptoms and progress, can help minimize the risk of complications and optimize recovery outcomes.

In addition to physical benefits, incorporating gentle movement and exercise into the rehabilitation process can also have positive effects on mental and emotional well-being. Physical activity releases endorphins, which are natural mood elevators, helping to reduce stress, anxiety, and depression commonly associated with the recovery period.

Overall, gentle movement and exercise are essential components of orthopedic surgery recovery, promoting physical rehabilitation, functional independence, and emotional well-being. By incorporating appropriate exercises into their daily routine and working closely with healthcare professionals, individuals can optimize their recovery outcomes and regain confidence in their ability to move and function effectively.

Stress Management Techniques for Overall Well-Being:
The recovery period following orthopedic surgery can be physically and emotionally challenging, often accompanied by stress, anxiety, and uncertainty about the future. Managing stress

effectively is essential for promoting overall well-being and optimizing the healing process.

There are various stress management techniques that individuals can incorporate into their daily routines to help cope with the challenges of recovery. Mindfulness meditation, deep breathing exercises, and progressive muscle relaxation are examples of relaxation techniques that can help reduce stress levels and promote a sense of calm and relaxation.

In addition to formal relaxation practices, engaging in enjoyable activities such as hobbies, creative pursuits, or spending time in nature can also help alleviate stress and promote emotional well-being. These activities provide a much-needed distraction from the challenges of recovery and can help individuals maintain a positive outlook on their healing journey.

Social support is another essential component of stress management during the recovery period.

Connecting with friends, family members, or support groups can provide emotional support, encouragement, and reassurance during difficult times. Sharing experiences with others who have undergone similar procedures can also offer valuable insights and perspectives.

Individuals need to prioritize self-care during the recovery process and make time for activities that nourish their body, mind, and spirit. This may include getting adequate rest, maintaining a healthy diet, staying hydrated, and practicing good hygiene habits.

Overall, stress management techniques play a crucial role in promoting overall well-being during orthopedic surgery recovery. By incorporating relaxation practices, engaging in enjoyable activities, and seeking social support, individuals can effectively cope with the challenges of recovery and cultivate resilience in the face of adversity.

Integrating Self-Care Into Your Recovery Routine:

Self-care is an essential aspect of the recovery process following orthopedic surgery, encompassing activities that promote physical, emotional, and mental well-being. Integrating self-care practices into your daily routine can help facilitate healing, reduce stress, and enhance overall quality of life during the recovery period.

One of the key components of self-care is prioritizing rest. Adequate sleep is essential for tissue repair, immune function, and overall recovery. Individuals need to establish a regular sleep routine, create a comfortable sleep environment, and practice relaxation techniques to promote restful sleep.

Nutrition is another critical aspect of self-care during the recovery process. Eating a balanced diet rich in nutrients, vitamins, and minerals is essential for supporting healing and optimizing recovery outcomes. Individuals need to stay hydrated, eat regular meals, and incorporate a variety of fruits, vegetables, lean proteins, and whole grains into their diet.

Physical activity is also an essential component of self-care, as it promotes strength, flexibility, and overall well-being.

Engaging in gentle exercises, such as walking, swimming, or yoga, can help improve circulation, reduce stiffness, and enhance mood during the recovery period.

In addition to physical self-care, individuals need to prioritize their emotional and mental well-being during the recovery process. This may involve engaging in activities that promote relaxation, stress management, and emotional expression, such as journaling, meditation, or therapy.

Self-care also encompasses advocating for your needs and seeking support when necessary. Individuals need to communicate openly with their healthcare team, ask questions, and seek clarification about their treatment plan and recovery process. Seeking support from friends, family members, or support groups can also provide valuable encouragement and reassurance during difficult times.

Overall, integrating self-care practices into your recovery routine is essential for promoting healing, reducing stress, and enhancing overall well-being during the orthopedic surgery recovery process.

By prioritizing rest, nutrition, physical activity, and emotional well-being, individuals can optimize their recovery outcomes and cultivate resilience in the face of adversity.

CONCLUSION

embarking on the journey of post-bariatric surgery recovery demands a comprehensive approach that extends far beyond mere dietary adjustments.

The insights shared in this guide underscore the importance of holistic healing, weaving together nutritional strategies, practical meal plans, and wellness tips to unlock the secrets to post-bariatric surgery success.

From laying the nutritional foundations for healing to preparing your kitchen as a sanctuary for recovery, each chapter has been meticulously crafted to provide invaluable guidance.

We've explored nourishing breakfasts, healing soups, and easy-to-digest main courses, all designed to support your body's needs during this critical phase.

Moreover, we've delved into the significance of hydration, the role of special considerations for orthopedic surgery recovery, and the incorporation of holistic healing practices beyond the plate.

These insights underscore the interconnectedness of body, mind, and spirit in the journey towards optimal health and wellness.

As you navigate through this transformative period, remember that patience, consistency, and self-compassion are your greatest allies. By embracing the principles outlined in this comprehensive guide and cultivating a mindful approach to your recovery journey, you're not just nourishing your body – you're nourishing your spirit, paving the way for a future filled with vitality, resilience, and boundless well-being.